Attention Deficit Hyperactivity Disorder Or ADHD Explained

Types, Diagnosis, Symptoms, Treatment, Causes, Neurocognitive Disorders, Prognosis, Research, History, Myths, and More!

By Frederick Earlstein

Foreword

Symptoms of hyperactivity have been observed in children from as early as the 19th century, and yet ADHD still remains to be one of the most controversial mental disorders today. As many as 39 million people as of 2013, according to the World Health Organization, and 30-50% of children diagnosed continue to experience the symptoms of ADHD well into adulthood. And yet we still do not know much about this condition. Its very existence has been questioned by many people, and there are those who still refuse to believe that it is a real mental disorder.

The fact of the matter is that we simply do not know enough about ADHD - its causes, how it works, its effects, and why it affects certain individuals and not others. Perhaps the only thing that experts can agree on at this point is that it is a very real disorder, with very severe and long-lasting effects on people's lives. It is to be hoped that as our knowledge and understanding of this condition grows, so will our acceptance of it, and our capacity to provide the proper treatments to those suffering from ADHD.

Table of Contents

Introduction

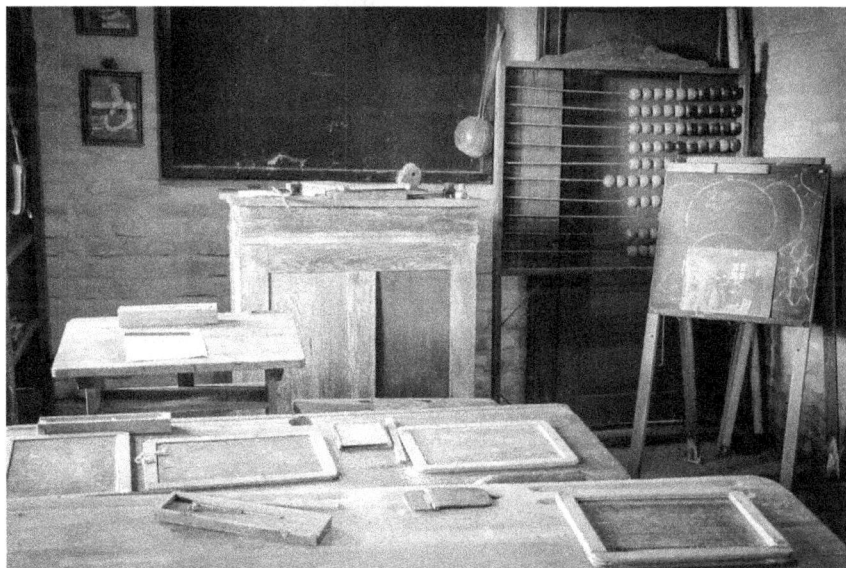

What differentiates a stubborn and misbehaving child from a child suffering from ADHD? This is perhaps the crux of the matter in our understanding of ADHD - that it is not simply a matter of child rebellion, stubbornness, or inability to apply themselves - despite the fact that the symptoms are very similar to children who are simply being difficult. The difference is that there are biological differences in the brain chemistry and functions among those who suffer from ADHD - which means that they cannot help themselves. The part of the brain responsible for control, behavior, emotions, movement, etc. - mainly located in the frontal lobes - are compromised. They are not functioning as well as one should expect in a person without ADHD.

This is just one of the recent developments in the field of research regarding ADHD. In this book, we bring together some of the widely accepted facts, opinions, and theories regarding ADHD that is prevalent in the medical and scientific community today. It is hoped that early recognition, identification, and treatment of this condition can provide people with ADHD with the means to cope with the struggles of their daily lives - a feat made more difficult by the unique symptoms of ADHD.

Important Terms to Know

ADD - Attention Deficit Disorder, an older term for ADHD

ADHD - Attention Deficit Hyperactivity Disorder, the official name given this condition by the American Psychiatric Association's Diagnostic and Statistical Manual of Mental Disorders.

Co-existing conditions - When two or more health conditions are present in the same individual (also, co-morbid)

Executive Function Deficit - When people with ADHD have difficulty in executive functions, or in the skills that help them start and finish a task.

Multimodal Treatment - A comprehensive approach to treatment in children, including multiple interventions working together, tailored to the child's unique individual needs.

Neurotransmitter - A chemical in the brain that acts as a messenger to help transmit nerve impulses between brain cells.

Non-stimulant medication - Medication approved to treat ADHD, but which is not classified by the FDA as a "controlled substance."

Rebound effect - A tendency in some medications to lead to symptoms of greater severity after being withdrawn from use. The effect may or may not be temporary.

Stimulant Medication - The most approved medication treatment for ADHD, and works by "stimulating" certain activities in the body's nervous system. When taken as prescribed, these can improve ADHD symptoms by promoting alertness, awareness, and the individual's ability to focus.

Chapter One: What is ADHD?

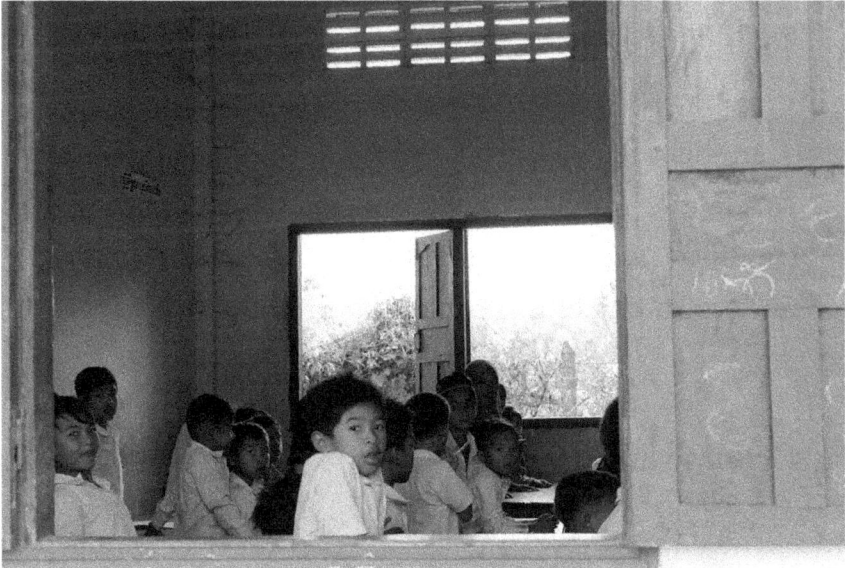

It was only with the publications of the several editions of the American Pychiatric Association's (APA's) Diagnostic and Statistical Manual of Mental Disorders (DSM) that ADHD (as we know it today has been officially recognized as a mental disorder. With each successive edition, the definition, the name, the types and the diagnosis of ADHD has been continually refined based on our growing body of information regarding this condition. It is not at all unexpected to find more changes being proposed in the scientific and medical community regarding definitions, types, impact, diagnosis, and even the treatment of ADHD in the years to come. It seems that as with anything else, the first hurdle had been acceptance of ADHD's legitimacy as a real mental disorder.

In this chapter, we take a look at the current definition of ADHD, the myths and misconceptions surrounding this condition, and the evolution of our knowledge and understanding of this condition throughout the years.

Defining ADHD

ADHD stands for Attention Deficit Hyperactivity Disorder, and it is considered a mental disorder of the neurodevelopmental or neurobehavioral type - or how the brain affects our emotions, behavior and learning. Starting at around the ages of 6-12, it is characterized by persistent behavioral problems in attention, hyperactivity, and impulsivity. When present for more than 6 months, and when it causes problems in at least two settings, then it is generally considered as falling under the ambit of ADHD.

This is a chronic condition affecting millions of children in the world - some 39 million people, according to statistics by the World Health Organization (WHO) in 2013. And while symptoms do seem to lessen with age, some 30-50% continue having symptoms well into adulthood.

Now, as always, and similar to the state of medical and expert opinions before ADHD became recognized as a medical disorder, the opinions regarding diagnosis of ADHD diverge widely. Some feel that it is over-diagnosed, while others feel it is under-diagnosed and under-treated. What does seem certain is that the number of children being diagnosed with ADHD has risen. Though this may just be due to the evolution and expansion of the coverage of ADHD, and because of greater public awareness of this condition.

Myths and Misconceptions about ADHD

ADHD is a condition replete with myths, misconceptions, and even stereotypes - from those questioning the very existence of ADHD as a valid disorder, to those who think that ADHD is simply a benign condition that is being excessively over-diagnosed. Certainly, no one can deny that the fast-paced, competitive and stressful environment within which children are now being raised could very well lead to misdiagnosis and mislabeling of children as having ADHD. Does this mean that ADHD is not a real medical condition? Of course not. There are many individuals who do suffer from ADHD, and yet who must also suffer the negative public perception and stigma that is attached to being diagnosed with this disorder - including the mistaken notion that it is not a real disorder at all.

While the basic elements of ADHD such as definitions and categories or types may be straightforward in itself - the myths, misconceptions, and public perceptions regarding ADHD are not quite so difficult to penetrate. Perhaps it has something to do with each family's traditional or personal parenting styles, and with the universal notion that while any child may misbehave, a child's behavior and discipline is the responsibility of the parents. When experts step in to say that these children can't help themselves from misbehaving, it is completely valid for parents to wonder whether the ADHD label really helps or actually harms their own children, by giving them an excuse for not adhering to proper discipline and behavior. But where should the line be drawn?

In this section, we take a closer look at some of the most prevalent myths and misconceptions regarding ADHD, and in doing so, perhaps gain a better understanding of this condition.

- *That having ADHD means that you're hyperactive.* Not necessarily. ADHD is characterized by ongoing patterns of either inattention, hyperactivity-impulsivity, or a combination of both. Inattention - by which a person lacks persistence, has difficulty sustaining his focus, is disorganized, and wanders off tasks - and when these problems are not due to defiance of lack of comprehension, can be sufficient for a diagnosis of ADHD.

- *That ADHD is not a real disorder.* There is a general consensus among international experts in the field that ADHD is, in fact, a valid disorder with severe and lifelong consequences - with a strong negative impact on practically every aspect of an individual's life until well into adulthood. Children diagnosed with ADHD are more likely to suffer from other psychiatric disorders and to require medical and emergency treatments; are more likely to drop out of school and to engage in antisocial activities in adolescence; and to suffer from depression and employment difficulties during adulthood. The problem then is very real, and its effects are quite serious and life-altering.

- *That ADHD only affects children.* A majority (70-80%) of children diagnosed with ADHD still struggle with its symptoms and manifestations until well into adulthood - including a higher risk for associated psychiatric disorders, as well as social isolation or rejection. Many times, it may seem like the child has "outgrown" ADHD, when in reality, the symptoms just seem different - for instance, what seems like diminished hyperactivity may only be a mask for an inner restlessness and need for activity. Or it may simply be that the individual had a different type of ADHD - inattention, for instance, other than hyperactivity. The symptom of inattention, on the other hand, is still quite present among many adults, and far more debilitating now because of the many different organizational tasks that adults are expected to be responsible for.
- *That poor parenting causes ADHD.* While we stil aren't sure what causes ADHD, and while environmental factors such as poor parenting can

contribute or exacerbate ADHD, studies have already found that the cause of ADHD cannot be ascribed exclusively to social factors. Genetic factors account for at least 80 percent of the variance of ADHD symptoms - greater than environmental factors. In fact, these factors (such as exposure to environmental toxins, allergic reactions of certain foods, family problems and marital discord, ineffective discipline, lack of motivation, educational or occupational status, or lazy learning habits, etc.) were not found to have a significant contribution to the development of ADHD symptoms. These inaccurate or "false" beliefs which attributed the ADHD symptoms to the children themselves (that the children can control their symptoms and that their behavior is therefore intentional) did contribute to comorbid disorders and only served to compromise or complicate treatment effectiveness.

- *That ADHD is over-diagnosed and over-medicated.* Actually, according to some, some children with ADHD may actually be undiagnosed and untreated. When legislation was passed in the 1990s that increased general awareness of ADHD, and prescribed the legal basis for its diagnosis and treatment in the school setting, the number of children diagnosed with ADHD did increase - as well as the school-based services available to them. The general opinion is that these developments may have led some to conclude that ADHD is over-diagnosed. And while prescriptions for the leading stimulant medication for hyperactivity (Ritalin) has certainly increased, many simply ascribe this to the growing awareness and better diagnosis tools we have of identifying this condition. When prescribed, physicians tend to use less than the optimal doses, and the overall rate of medication and stimulant use among school-age children is still relatively low - 2.8% of elementary-age children, and 99% of whom use stimulants of the prescribed medication. The truth is that claims of over-diagnosis and over-medication is still difficult to prove.

- *That ADHD stimulant medication leads to addiction.* There is simply no data to back up this claim. In fact, according to recent studies, people with ADHD who take stimulant medication tend to have lower rates of substances abuse than people with ADHD who don't take medication. On the other hand, no causative link has been found in a long-term study comparing childhood and early teen use of stimulant medication and the incidence of the use of drugs, alcohol, or nicotine among early adult males with ADHD.

- *That ADHD isn't a big deal, or that people with ADHD just don't "want" to focus - they just need to try harder.* Having ADHD isn't a matter of simply wanting to do something, and willing oneself to do it. People with ADHD have to struggle just to get the simple things right - and this struggle could prevail in all areas of their life, for their entire lifetime. ADHD is a big deal when you consider its broad range of negative effects - from job performance, employment status, family and social relationships, or just doing simple things like paying the bills on time, buying groceries, locking the door. This is why proper diagnosis and treatment of ADHD is important - imagine the difference between a person with ADHD struggling and trying harder than everyone else their entire lives, as opposed to a person with ADHD who has the benefit of ADHD coping strategies and treatment to aid him in these daily tasks and activities.
- *That boys are more likely to have ADHD than girls.* Both boys and girls can be diagnosed with ADHD -

the difference, perhaps, is in the type of symptoms they tend to have. Girls may tend to internalize more compared to boys, and may have lower hyperactivity rates and conduct problems than the boys - which would probably explain why girls have lower referral rates. This does not mean, however, that the severity is less pronounced in girls: according to a 1999 study, girls were more likely to have issues on substance abuse, alcohol, drug and cigarette use, and were at a higher risk for panic and obsessive compulsive disorders. In fact, girls may be more affected by environmental factors than the boys. This makes long-term and further studies into ADHD diagnosis and treatment methods very important.

History of ADHD

The term Attention Deficit Hyperactivity Disorder (ADHD) was coined fairly recently - in 1987, but the condition itself – or similar conditions of hyperactivity - have been recognized from as early as the 18th century, or over the past 200 years. Below is a brief timeline of the evolution of what we know of this condition:

- In 1775, prominent German physician Melchior Adam Weikard published a textbook called *Der Philosophische Arzt*, which contained what might possibly be considered the first medical description of ADHD-like behavior. Most of the terms used are pretty general: inattentive, shallow, superficial, reckless, and treating everything in a light manner." Interestingly, the treatment prescribed by Weikard includes being kept solitary when he is too active, and "rubbing, cold baths, steep powder, chinchona, mineral waters, horseback riding, and gymnastic exercises."

- In 1789, Sir Alexander Crichton, a Scottish born physician and author wrote a book entitled *An Inquiry into the Nature and Origin of Mental Derangement*, which also contained detailed descriptions of a mental condition similar to ADHD, which he referred to as a "disease of inattention" or what was more commonly referred to by people as "the fidgets." It is theorized that a possible association with Weikard (Crichton received medical training in Germany, in several areas where Weikard practiced medicine) may have led or guided him to these observations, but Crichton's descriptions were a lot more detailed.

Thus, the "incapability of attending with constancy to any one object..." may "either be born with a person or the effect of an accidental disease." Children who suffered from this condition, according to Crichton, needed special educational intervention.

- In 1844, German physician Heinrich Hoffman created an illustrated storybook "Struwwelpeter" as a Christmas present for his son. Hoffman often used drawings to calm and amuse crying children - these were later on published as "Cheerful Stories and Funny Pictures with 15 colored plates for children from 3 to 6 years" (1845). It was a successful book, and the following year, Hoffman came out with a second edition, with additional stories that now included "Fidgety Phil" (Zappelphilipp) - now a popular allegory for children with ADHD. In this story, Philip displays ADHD-like behavior such as persistent inattention, hyperactivity, and motoric overactivity over dinner - causing his falling over in his chair, pulling down the food on the table with him, and provoking the anger of his parents. As for most children with ADHD, the symptoms can cause significant impairment in social functioning. "Johnny Look-in-the-air" is the story of a boy showing severe inattention, always looking at the sky and clouds, until he collided with a dog and fell into a river." Yet again, another depiction of significant inattention that is similar to that of children suffering from ADHD. It seems likely, however, that Hoffman merely intended an illustrated children's book rather than a description of a pathological condition which, at the time, were not yet established as a psychiatric disorder. Nevertheless, Fidgety Phil has become one of the most commonly used allegory depicting the diagnostic criteria of ADHD.

- In 1902, Sir George Frederic Still gave a lecture to the Royal College of Physicians in London. He described 43 children with an "abnormal incapacity for sustained attention." Despite normal intellect, such children displayed aggressiveness, defiance, resistance to discipline, excessive emotions or passions, low inhibitions, and the seeming inability to learn from the consequences of their actions. For the first time, Still introduced the concept of moral defect, or a defect of moral consciousness that cannot be ascribed to an impairment of the intellect. He also postulated that the condition was caused by a biological predisposition that was hereditary or was the result of a pre- or post-natal injury.

- From 1917 to 1928, a worldwide epidemic of encephalitis lethargica affected approximately 20 million people around the world. Many of the affected children also showed residual abnormal behavior which were termed as "postencephalitic behavior disorder." This was a realistic case of what some authors have been saying since 1908: a correlation between early brain damage and subsequent behavior problems or learning difficulties. The actual behaviors observed among children included a significant change in personality, emotional instability, cognitive defects, learning difficulties, depression, poor motor control. They also became hyperactive, irritable, distractible, antisocial, destructive, unruly, and unmanageable. While not technically meeting the definitions of ADHD, this disorder nevertheless raised a broad interest in hyperactivity among children.

By the mid-20th century, various cases of this condition were often referred to by different names: "minimal brain damage," "minimal brain dysfunction," "minimal brain disorder," "learning/behavioral disabilities," or hyperactivity. As our knowledge of the condition grew, these terms became problematic as not being entirely accurate, or unified.

- In 1968, the Diagnostic and Statistical Manual of Mental Disorders (DSM-II) coined the term "Hyperkinetic Reaction of Childhood." But because hyperactivity was not always a factor, the term was refined to "Attention-Deficit Disorder (ADD) with or without hyperactivity" in 1980 by DSM III. In 1987, in DSM-III-R and subsequent editions, Attention Deficit Hyperactivity Disorder (ADHD) was used, but now with recognized subtypes, including the lack of a hyperactivity component. Today, more studies continue to be published as our knowledge of this condition grows.

Chapter Two: Types of ADHD

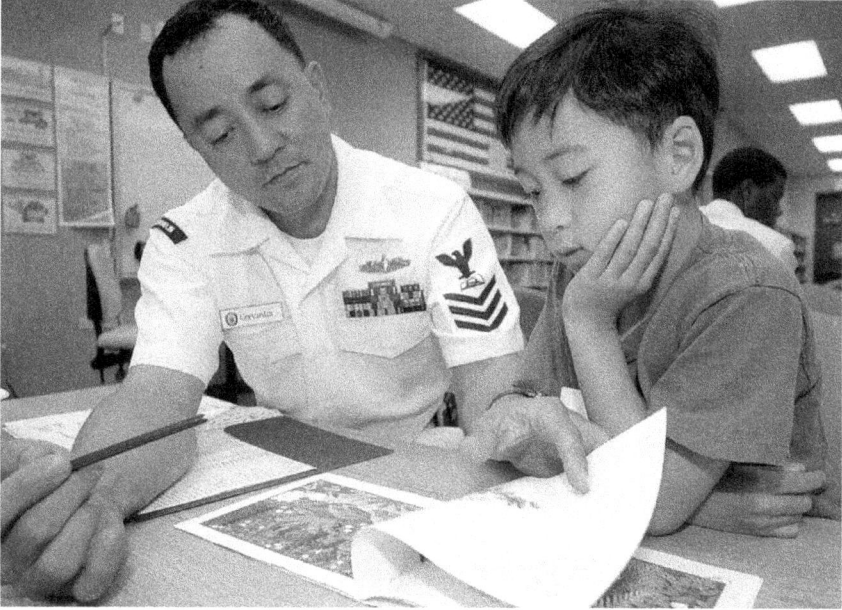

ADHD is divided into three different types, based primarily on the prominent or prevalent symptoms that a person has. Based on the definition of ADHD, there are three behavioral patterns that are affected among persons diagnosed with ADHD:

- Inattention - Disorganization, attention wanders off tasks, lacks persistence, difficulty sustaining focus - when these problems are not due to defiance or lack of comprehension. A person suffering from inattention gets distracted easily, has poor concentration and organizational skills.

- Hyperactivity - Constant movement, excessive fidgeting, tapping, or talking, even in situations where it is not appropriate. In adults, hyperactivity can be seen as extreme restlessness or constant activity. A hyperactive person never seems to slow down, is constantly talking and fidgeting, and has difficulty staying on task.

- Impulsivity - Hasty actions without forethought and which may have high potential for harm, or a desire for immediate rewards or inability to delay gratification. A person may also be socially intrusive, interrupts others excessively, or makes important decisions without considering long-term consequences.

The three types of ADHD are, therefore:

1. Predominantly inattentive;

2. Predominantly hyperactive-impulsive;

3. A combination thereof

It is important to note that not all individuals may experience or show these symptoms in the same way. The treatment that may eventually be deemed best for an individual will largely be based on the symptoms he or she has. Below we take a closer look at these three different types of ADHD.

Different types of ADHD

1. Predominantly Inattentive

A child diagnosed with a Predominantly Inattentive Type of ADHD has difficulty focusing or concentrating. While most children can have moments of inattention, and dreamer-type children can often be found staring out a window, lost in thought, this does not necessarily mean that they have ADHD. To constitute the inattentive type of ADHD, the child's symptoms are more severe and causes more difficulty for them in their daily functions as compared to children with normal bouts of inattention.

In the Predominantly Inattentive-type of ADHD, an individual may be disorganized, is easily distracted, has trouble prioritizing, and has difficulty starting and finishing tasks. They can have trouble concentrating even while reading something. This inability to stay focused can have a negative impact on their ambitions, relationships, school or work goals, and careers.

2. Predominantly Hyperactive-Impulsive

In contrast to the Predominantly Inattentive Type, individuals with the Predominantly Hyperactive-Impulsive Type of ADHD are, as the name suggests, characterized by hyperactivity and impulsivity. Although they may also display symptoms of inattention, these are not as marked or as predominant as the symptoms of hyperactivity and impulsivity.

These individuals can be quite disruptive in a learning setting such as a school. And similar to the Inattentive Type ADHD, the hyperactivity has to be more extreme than that of most normal, high-energy children. It is a very real kind of restlessness and a need for constant activity or motion. The type of hyperactivity and impulsivity which constitutes ADHD will cause very real problems in a child's life - including difficulty learning, difficulty in social situations when they speak out of turn, talk too much, interrupt other people, are socially intrusive, or are easily bored. They may engage in an activity or make major decisions without first considering long-term consequences, or the potential for harm.

3. Combination

The Combination Type ADHD among individuals usually means an almost coequal manifestation of the symptoms of both inattentive and hyperactive-impulsive type ADHD. This is actually considered to be the most common type of ADHD, as most individuals diagnosed with ADHD usually show symptoms of both types at one point or another.

Seven Types of ADHD by Dr. Daniel Amen

Interestingly, psychiatrist Dr. Daniel Amen has recently proposed 7 different types of ADHD, as opposed to the 3 conventional types. He built on work started in the 1980s by Joel Lubar, PhD, who found that children and teenagers with ADD had decreased brain activity during concentration. Normal brain response usually shows faster or increased brain wave activity during concentration, but Lubar's research showed slower brain waves in the frontal lobes. This was followed by 1990 findings by Dr. Alan Zametkin that showed significant brain underactivity in the prefrontal cortex of people with ADHD in response to an intellectual challenge. Normally, one expects an increase, rather than a decrease in brain activity during periods of concentration or intellectual problems. To bolster these findings, they also found a significant underproduction and unavailability of dopamine in the brain.

Based on some 100,000 SPECT brain imaging scans, Dr. Amen isolated 7 different types of ADHD. His theory is that the more narrowly you can target a person's ADHD type, the more effective the treatment can be.

Dr. Amen's 7 types of ADHD is still controversial - some call it ground-breaking, while others are more skeptical. It still remains to be seen, however, whether or not these 7 types of ADHD will be accepted by the medical and psychiatric community, and to what extent the proposed treatments will prove effective. In the interests of objectivity, however, we present you below with Dr. Amen's 7 types of ADHD, along with a brief overview of each:

1. Classic ADD

Characterized by inattention, distractibility, hyperactivity, disorganization and impulsivity. Scans show decreased brain activity during concentration, as well as dopamine deficiency.

2. Inattentive ADD

Characterized by short attention spans, distractibility, disorganization, and procrastination and daydreaming. Scans show low activity in the prefrontal cortex, and dopamine deficiency. Affects girls more than boys, and does not show hyperactivity or impulsivity.

3. Overfocused ADD

Overfocused ADD is characterized by the core symptoms of Classic ADD, including trouble shifting attention and getting stuck in negative thought patterns or behaviors. Scans show dopamine and serotonin deficiencies, as well as over-activity in the anterior cingulate gyrus.

4. Temporal Lobe ADD

Temporal Lobe ADD is characterized by the core symptoms of ADD, including learning, memory, and behavioral problems such as anger, aggression, and mild paranoia. Scans show abnormalities in the temporal lobe, as well as decreased activity in the prefrontal cortex.

5. Limbic ADD

Characterized by the core symptoms of Classic ADD, including chronic low-level sadness, moodiness, low energy, feelings of helplessness or excessive guilt, and chronic low self-esteem. Scans show too much activity in the limbic part of the brain and decreased prefrontal cortex activity.

6. Ring of Fire ADD

Characterized by sensivity to noise, light, and touch. There may be periods of mean, nasty behavior, unpredictability, fast speaking, anxiety, and fearfulness. Scans show a ring of hyperactivity around the brain (where the entire brain is overactive).

7. Anxious ADD

Characterized by the core symptoms of ADD, as well as anxiety, tension, symptoms of physical stress such as headaches and stomachaches, and a freezing response during anxiety-provoking situations. Scans show high activity in the basal ganglia.

Dr. Daniel Amen works from The Amen Clinics. If you are interested in finding out more about his work on the 7 types of ADD, you can visit his website here:

Attention Deficit Disorder ADD/ADHD:
<http://danielamenmd.com/healthy-vs-unhealthy-2/attention-deficit-disorder-addadhd/>

Chapter Three: Causes of ADHD

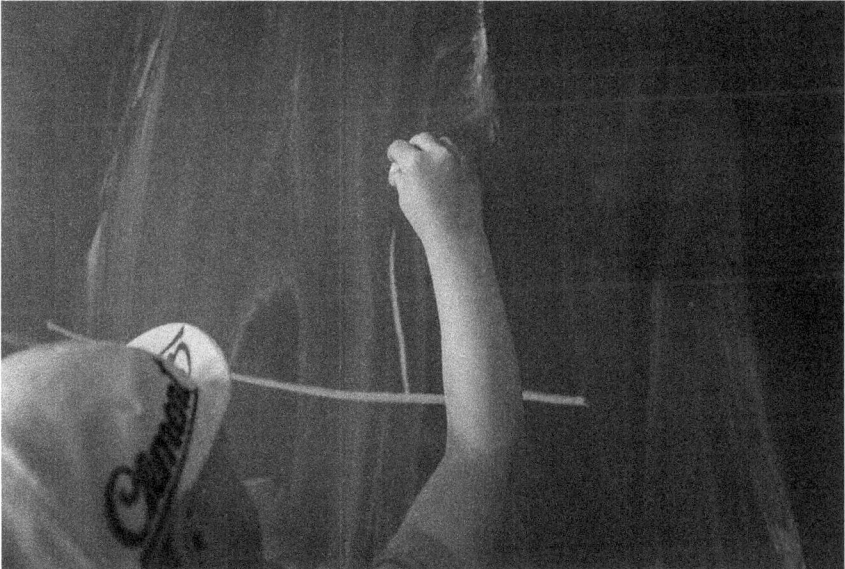

While we cannot yet pinpoint with any level of certainty what the precise cause or causes of ADHD are, studies have at least narrowed down the possible causes to interactions between both genetic and environmental factors. It has also been determined that trauma or infection to the brain may lead to ADHD. But there is no single cause that is solely responsible for ADHD.

What scientists do agree on is that ADHD is a medical disorder that affects different areas of the brain, especially the frontal area. This area is mostly responsible for functions such as memory, thinking, planning, organizing, and the regulation or control of behavior. The factors that can influence the brain's functions include heredity and external factors such as exposure to toxic substances, and brain injury, trauma or disease.

In this chapter, based on information from the most recent research available, we take a closer look at the possible causes of ADHD, as well as factors that have already been disproved as having causative links to ADHD. What is apparent is that ADHD is not caused by factors within the child's control - such as laziness, poor motivation, low intelligence, or poor upbringing. If anything, there seems to be a biological component to ADHD which bolsters the fact that this is a very real mental disorder.

Brain Chemistry

Recent studies have shown that ADHD may be the result of an imbalance of at least two chemical messengers, or neurotransmitters, in the brain, particularly in the prefrontal cortex, which is the area of the brain responsible for attention, behavior, judgment, and emotional responses. When neutrotransmitters are not in balance, regions of the prefrontal cortex may not function properly, resulting in behavior such as inattention, hyperactivity or impulsivity.

And while the significance to ADHD has not yet been shown, analysis of brain imaging scans of those affected with ADHD showed 3-4 percent smaller brain volumes in all brain regions - the frontal lobe, temporal gray matter, caudate nucleus, and cerebellum, as well as an abnormally small volume of white matter. Interestingly, children with ADHD who were on medication had white matter volume similar to those of unaffected children.

Lower levels of Dopamine may also play a role. This is a brain chemical that carries signals between nerves in the brain, and is linked to mood, attention, learning, sleep, and movement.

Genetics

ADHD frequently runs in families. Sometimes, a parent and a child are diagnosed with ADHD at the same time. This does not mean, however, that all children in a family will have ADHD.

Genetics has been found as a causative factor in the majority of ADHD cases - often, a child with ADHD is four times more likely to have had a relative also diagnosed with this disorder. Anywhere from a third to a half of parents with ADHD are more likely to have a child with this disorder. Genetic characteristics seem to be passed down, but the precise genetic cause has yet to be isolated.

Environmental Factors

Various factors in the environment may also increase the risk of the development of ADHD, whether these took place during pregnancy, delivery, infancy, or during a child's developmental years.

Toxins in the Environment

For instance, lead in the body may affect a child's development and behavior - this was suggested back when lead components were found in paint used in homes prior to 1978. But although lead is no longer used as a component of paint, children who live in older buildings may still be exposed to toxic levels of lead from old paint.

Pesticides may also play a role in the risks of developing ADHD.

Prenatal Exposure

Substances such as alcohol or nicotine may increase the risk of the child developing ADHD. Maternal smoking may have a link to ADHD, but because women who suffer from ADHD are also more likely to smoke, the genetic factor may also be the determining factor. Nicotine can, however, cause hypoxia (lack of oxygen) in utero.

Pregnancy Problems

Difficulties during the pregnancy, children born premature or with a low birth weight, are also at a higher risk of developing ADHD.

Brain Injuries, Trauma, Brain Tumors, Strokes, or Disease

Brain injury may cause ADHD-like symptoms in individuals previously without this disorder - mainly due to frontal lobe damage.

In a small number of children, it was also found that brain injury following exposure to toxins or physical injury may also cause attention deficit disorder.

Overall, however, only a small percentage of children with ADHD were found to have suffered from brain injury or trauma.

Other possible causes of brain injury that may lead to ADHD include brain tumors, a stroke, or a disease.

Disproved Causes of ADHD

It is easy to suddenly begin suspecting many things in the environment of having a hand in the development of a child's ADHD, but sometimes such fears are only that - fears with little evidence in fact. The following, for instance, have not been linked to ADHD:

● Food additives, sugar, and allergies

This is one of the more popular theories regarding the cause of a child's behavior - their diet and nutrition, especially when they have had too much sugar or food additives, have been pinpointed as a possible cause of ADHD behavior.

But while it has yet to be found whether or not sugar contributes or exacerbates ADHD symptoms, sugar itself has not been isolated as a cause of ADHD. In short, simply removing sugar from a child's diet is unlikely to impact significantly on ADHD behavior.

By this same token, there was no evidence to show any significant link between ADHD and an individual's allergies to specific food substances.

Targeting nutrition may, however, help alleviate ADHD behavior. For instance, the lack of or a deficiency of Omega-3 fatty acids may actually contribute to ADHD development. Omega-3 fatty acids are considered important for brain development and brain functions, and when given as supplements, it may help to alleviate symptoms in some children, and in some cases, have even helped to boost school performance.

● Parenting or child rearing

Many parents may look to themselves as to the possible cause of ADHD in children - whether it is in their parenting methods or child rearing techniques. The common tendency is to look to the parents, and indeed bad parenting and dysfunctional family dynamics may contribute to ADHD-like symptoms among children.

But the truth is that there is simply not enough evidence linking parenting or child rearing techniques to ADHD, and not enough to isolate this as a possible cause. Not all children who grow up and are raised in the same environment will develop ADHD. Other factors, whether genetic, or environmental causes that also impact a child's physiological development, seem to be more likely causes of ADHD.

- Hormones

No studies have shown any significant connection between ADHD and hormonal problems or hormone functioning.

- Watching too much TV

Neither was any link found between ADHD and watching too much TV. Nor is there any indication that children with ADHD watch more television than those who do not have ADHD.

Chapter Four: Symptoms and Diagnosis of ADHD

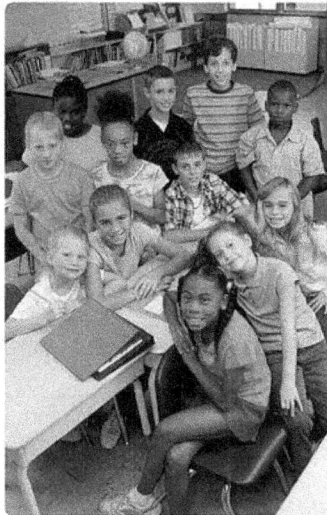

FDA *Consumer Health Information*
www.fda.gov/consumer

How Do You Know If Your Child Has ADHD?

Is your child in constant motion? Does he or she talk incessantly? Or have trouble focusing and prefer to daydream?

Then your child may have attention deficit hyperactivity disorder, or ADHD.

This childhood disorder often begins between the ages of 3 and 6 years, according to the National Institute of Mental Health (NIMH). And it may continue through the teenage years and into adulthood.

Three types of ADHD are recognized:
- inattentive (trouble focusing, following instructions, and finishing tasks)
- hyperactive-impulsive (constantly on the go, talking excessively, and interrupting others)
- combined (symptoms of both inattention and hyperactivity-impulsivity)

Diagnosis

Studies show that the number of children being diagnosed with ADHD is increasing, and boys are more than twice as likely as girls to have it. According to the Centers for Disease Control and Prevention, as of 2007, about 9.5 percent of children 4 to 17 years old have at one time been diagnosed with ADHD.

Mark Ritter, M.D., R.Ph., who reviews drugs to treat ADHD at the Food and Drug Administration (FDA), explains the increase may be due to a greater public awareness of the disorder and psychiatric illnesses in general. And boys are more likely to have

1 / FDA Consumer Health Information / U.S. Food and Drug Administration   NOVEMBER 2011

The process by which a child might be diagnosed with ADHD involves several steps, from an analysis of the symptoms over a period of time, the age of onset, the effect on the child's immediate environment, and the ruling out of other possible causes of the symptoms.

While doctors and psychologists have observed tendencies towards hyperactivity, inattention, and impulsivity among certain children since the nineteenth century, it wasn't until the American Psychiatric Association's (APA) second edition of the Diagnostic and Statistical Manual of Mental Disorders (DSM) was published in 1968 that "hyperkinetic impulse disorder" was recognized for the first time. With subsequent editions, (DSM-III in 1980), the definitions, terminologies, and diagnostic criteria has continually been refined as scientists and experts discovered more about this condition.

In 1987, the name "Attention Deficit Hyperactivity Disorder (ADHD)" was first used. In the fourth edition of DSM in 2000, the three subtypes of ADHD was established, and is still used by healthcare professionals today. Further refinements were made in the most recent DSM-5TM, which was published in 2013. In this section, we will look at the most recent diagnostic tools for ADHD, based on the APA's 5th Edition DSM.

It must also be noted that while people with ADHD do tend to have lower scores in Intelligence Quotient (IQ) tests, this does not necessarily mean that people with ADHD are less intelligent. Because of symptoms of ADHD such as distractibility and inattention, it is difficult to determine a person's level of intelligence as divorced from the influence of the symptoms that they are experiencing.

An Overview of the DSM-5 Medical Classification System for ADHD

According to the APA's DSM-5, the following factors must be present to meet a diagnosis of ADHD:

1. A persistent pattern of inattention and/or hyperactivity-impulsivity that interferes with functioning or development, where six or more symptoms have persisted for at least six months. These must be inconsistent with developmental levels and must negatively impact social and academic/occupational activities.

2. Several of the symptoms of inattention or hyperactivity-impulsivity must have been present prior to the age of 12. This is the age of onset, and it is not necessary that the symptoms be shown to create any significant impairment - just that they be present.

3. Several of the symptoms of inattention or hyperactivity-impulsivity are present in at least two or more settings. This is called the multiple settings requirement.

4. A clear evidence that the symptoms interfere with, or reduce the quality of, social, academic, or occupational functions.

5. That the symptoms do not occur exclusively during the course of schizophrenia or other psychotic disorders, and are not better explained by another mental disorder (e.g., mood disorder, anxiety disorder, dissociative disorder, or a personality disorder).

Symptoms of Inattention and/or Hyperactivity-Impulsivity

DSM-5 goes on to enumerate the different symptoms of ADHD, both both for inattention and hyperactivity-impulsivity types of ADHD. Again, there must be at least six or more symptoms of either inattention or hyperactivity-impulsivity that are inappropriate for the individual's developmental level, and have been present for at least 6 months. This is true of children up to the age of sixteen. The criteria for adolescents and adults, or those age seventeen and above, DSM-5 prescribes at least five or more symptoms instead of six, though all other standards are the same. This latter change is on account of a lower symptom threshold for a reliable diagnosis in adults.

These are the following:

Inattention

- Often fails to give close attention to details or makes careless mistakes in schoolwork, at work, or with other activities.

- Often has trouble holding their attention on tasks or play activities.

- Often does not seem to listen when spoken to directly.

- Is often forgetful in daily activities.

- Is often easily distracted.

- Often does not follow through on instructions and fails to finish schoolwork, chores, or duties (loss of focus, easily side-tracked)

- Often has trouble organizing tasks and activities.

- Often avoids dislikes, or is reluctant to do tasks that require mental effort over a long period of time

- Often loses things necessary for tasks and activities.

Hyperactivity-Impulsivity

- Often fidgets with or taps hands or feet, or squirms in their seat.

- Often leaves their seat in situations where remaining seated is expected.

- Often interrupts or intrudes on others (e.g., butts into conversations)

- Often has trouble waiting his/her turn

- Often runs about or climbs in inappropriate situations (or a feeling of restlessness among adolescents or adults)

- Often unable to quietly play or to take part in leisure activities.

- Is often "on the go" or acting as if they were "driven by a motor"

- Often talks excessively

- Often blurts out an answer before a question has been completed.

Depending on which symptoms are present, a child may be be either predominantly inattentive, predominantly hyperactive-impulsive, or shows a combined type of ADHD. This is referred to as the "Presentations of ADHD." What is interesting is that because symptoms may also change over time, then the presentation may also change.

Classification based on Severity

DSM-5 also classifies ADHD based on the severity of the symptoms. Thus, one can have either mild, moderate, or severe ADHD:

1. Mild

The ADHD is mild when there are few, if any, symptoms in excess of the 5-6 symptoms needed for a diagnosis, are present. The effects are also no more than minor impairments in the individual's social or occupational functioning.

2. Moderate

The ADHD is Moderate if the symptoms and the functional impairment fall between Mild and Severe.

3. Severe

The ADHD is Severe if there are many or several symptoms present in addition to those required to make a diagnosis, and there is marked impairment in social or occupational functioning.

Associated Disorders

The onset or manifestation of the symptoms of ADHD may also appear alongside other problems or conditions. This may not always be the case, but seeing these associated conditions may be telling, and certainly does not exclude, the possibility of an ADHD diagnosis.

In children, for instance, ADHD often occurs with other disorders some 2/3 of the time. Some of the commonly associated conditions with ADHD in children include:

- Learning disabilities such as dyslexia

- Tourette Syndrome

- Oppositional Defiant Disorder (ODD) and Conduct Disorder (CD) which manifest as antisocial behaviors such as stubbornness, aggression, deceitfulness, lying, temper tantrums, and stealing.

- Primary disorder of vigilance, characterized by poor attention and concentration, and difficulty in staying awake.

- Anxiety Disorder

- Depression

- Sleep problems such as insomnia

- Autistic Spectrum Disorder (ASD) which affect social interaction, communication, interests, and behavior

- Epilepsy

- Mood disorders such as bipolar disorder and major depressive disorder

- Obsessive-compulsive disorder (OCD)

- Disorders involving substance use

- Restless Legs Syndrome

- Persistent bed wetting

On the other hand, among adults, the symptoms of ADHD may prove more difficult to isolate and identify. What is known is that among those diagnosed with ADHD as children, symptoms can and do still persist well into adulthood, whether a full range of symptoms, or in a diminished form or intensity. The way that inattentiveness, hyperactivity and impulsivity is simply different in its effects among adults as compared to the effects on children.

Hyperactivity, for instance, tends to decrease in adults, while inattentiveness tends to get worse due to the pressures of adult life and responsibilities.

The following are possible symptoms associated with ADHD in adults:

- Carelessness and lack of attention to detail

- Poor organizational skills

- Continually starting new tasks before finishing old ones

- Forgetfulness

- Restlessness and edginess

- Inability to focus or prioritize

- Continually losing or misplacing things

- Speaking out of turn and difficulty keeping quiet

- Mood swings, irritability and a quick temper

- Inability to deal with stress

- Blurting out responses and interrupting others

- Extreme impatience

- Taking risks, with little to no regard for personal safety or the safety of others.

- Difficulty in finding and staying in a job

- Difficulties in relationships, social interactions, drugs, and crime

ADHD in adults may also appear alongside other disorders including:

- Bipolar Disorder or severe mood swings

- Personality Disorders

- Obsessive-Compulsive Disorders (OCD)

Chapter Five: Treatment and Management of ADHD

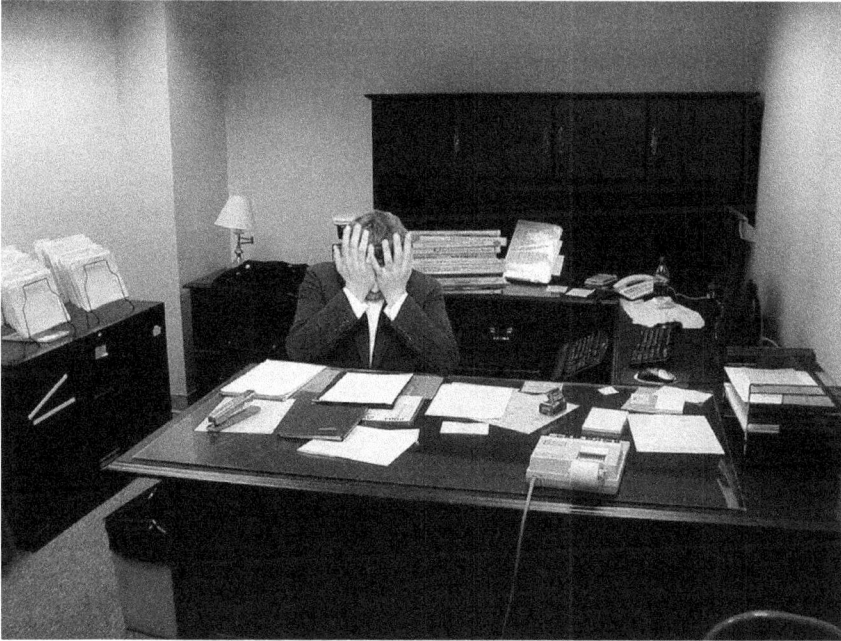

The usual and most accepted management of ADHD is medication and behavioral therapies or counseling - whether alone or in combination. Unfortunately, there is no such thing as a cure that would completely get rid of the negative symptoms of ADHD. Most of the treatment options available are geared mostly towards helping the individual manage the specific symptoms they are experiencing, while also providing them with useful skills or strategies to cope with the demands of daily life. Treatment and management, therefore, depend to a large extent on the symptoms each person experiences.

Medication

Please remember that all individuals, whether children or adults, inevitably respond differently to ADHD medication. If you are giving your child any ADHD medication, it is always a good idea to closely monitor any possible side-effects that your child may experience. Close coordination with your doctor is necessary in this case, as your consulting professional will need to adjust the dosage of the prescribed medication depending on the observed side-effects, if any. If you don't think that the medication is doing your child any good, or is not having any significant effects, don't hesitate to consult with your doctor about your intention of stopping or discontinuing medication. Work closely with your doctor as you slowly and gradually decrease the drugs until medication can safely be stopped altogether.

The guidelines on the use of ADHD medication varies by country, and are generally not recommended for preschool children. It is important that appropriate dosages by prescribed because underdosing may actually result in a lack of response or effectiveness later on. ADHD medication, whether stimulant or non-stimulant are generally safe - but they do have certain side-effects and contraindications, so these should not be taken or used indiscriminately.

Medical options for ADHD include Stimulant and non-Stimulant medication.

Stimulant Medication

This is considered the pharmaceutical treatment of choice, and have proven to be the most effective and are therefore the most commonly prescribed medication for ADHD, and are often prescribed in controlled-release methods. There are generally two kinds of stimulants: methylphenidate and amphetamine products. More specifically, these include:

- Substituted Phenethylamines such as Amphetamine and Methylphenidate (e.g., Ritalin Metadate, and Concerta)

- Dexmethylphenidate (e.g., Focalin)

- Dextroamphetamine (e.g., Dexedrine, Zenzedi)

- Mixed Amphetamine Salts (e.g., Adderall)

- Destroamphetamine (e.g., Desoxyn)

- Lisdexamfetamine (e.g., Vyvanse)

The effects of stimulant medication may vary, but usually runs the gamut of enhanced alertness, wakefulness, endurance, productivity, motivation, heart rate, blood pressure, and locomotion. These can also improve mood and relieve anxiety, with some even inducing feelings of euphoria. On the other hand, stimulant medication may also induce the perception of a diminished requirement for food and sleep, and some can also cause anxiety, hyperactivity, dysthmia, and potential heart failure when taken in high doses. Other possible side-effects of stimulants include headaches, stomachaches, insomnnia, decreased appetite, weight loss, nausea, and irritability.

Another potential side effect of the use of stimulant medication is that it may cause the body to significantly reduce the production of its own body chemicals that fulfill similar functions. A person coming off from the effects of a stimulant may also feel a "crash" that can include feelings of depression, lethargy, and confusion. The long-term effects of Stimulant Medication, however, has yet to be determined, though long-term misuse at extreme dosages may cause addiction and dependence. And yet, untreated ADHD may also lead to a higher risk of substance abuse and conduct disorders. Using stimulants appears to reduce this risk.

Non-Stimulant Medication

Certain non-stimulant medication may be used as an alternative ADHD medication, or added to stimulant therapy. Unfortunately, there are no significant studies showing the effects of non-stimulant medications on ADHD symptoms.

Antidepressants

While not specifically approved as ADHD treatments, antidepressants have been found to help with inattention, hyperactivity and impulsivity. They are at least an option for those diagnosed with ADHD, but who haven't been responding well to stimulants alone. They have been found to work well when ADHD symptoms take place alongside mood disorders such as depression or anxiety.

Behavioral Therapy or Behavioral Modification

Behavioral Therapy has been known to be quite a successful for children with ADHD. When done in concert with medication, the high effectivity of this type of treatment may allow you to reduce the dosage of prescribed stimulant medications.

In essence, Behavioral Therapy or Behavioral Modification involves the reinforcement of desired behaviors through rewards and praises, and decreasing the incidence of problem behaviors by setting limits and consequences.

The American Academy of Pediatrics has set three basic principles by which any behavioral therapy should be implemented:

1. Set specific goals

2. Provide rewards for desired behavior and consequences or unwanted results or for failing to meet a goal.

3. Long term use of rewards and consequences to help shape a child's behavior in a positive way

Any successful Behavioral Therapy or Behavioral Modification should be approached long-term. That is, handled with patience and with a view for long-term rather than short-term results. Children with ADHD may often prove variable in their behavior and it may be difficult to notice any success in behavioral therapies. Over time, however, behavioral therapy does help improve ADHD symptoms. That said, parents and family members also play an important part in Behavior Therapy, because they help reinforce any progress made in therapy in the home environment.

Social Skills Training

Some therapists do provide social skills training - and this can be invaluable to children diagnosed with ADHD, especially when their symptoms has them displaying undesirable social behavior such as controlling impulsive outbursts or avoiding interrupting others. To be truly successful, though, social skills training must eventually be translated into actual daily usage such as at home or in school.

Supporting Therapy in the Home Environment

In order to get the most out of any behavioral therapy or social skills training, it is important that the parents provide a supportive environment at home, where similar techniques may also be applied. To be able to do this successfully, parents must coordinate closely with their child's therapists in order to find what has been working well for their child's specific symptoms, and which techniques the therapists recommend they can implement at home.

For instance, rewards and praise, predictable routines, simplifying schedules, good organization at home, and creating a quiet place can be ways by which parents can create a consistent environment by which their child may learn behavioral modification techniques and coping strategies for ADHD symptoms. As with any form of training given a child - whether they have ADHD or nor - consistency and patience is key.

Some of the more specific ways by which parents and families can help support behavior therapy at home include:

- Limiting the child's choices to keep them from being overwhelmed

- Effective discipline such as the removal of privileges or timeouts rather than yelling or spanking

- Nurturing a healthy lifestyle, which includes a healthy and nutritious diet, plenty of physical activity and exercise, and sufficient sleep are natural yet effective ways to treat the symptoms of ADHD. And these are lifestyle choices and opportunities which can only be provided at home - not in a therapist's office.

- Create positive opportunities to encourage your child to do well, and reinforce these positive experiences with rewards and praise.

- Be brief, clear, and specific when communicating with your child. Avoid mixed messages, and use clear directions when you are giving them directions or guidance.

- Encourage organization - guide them in organizing their things, their clothing, toys, school bag, and other stuff to keep down incidence of forgetfulness or misplacing important items.

- Provide them with a clean, distraction-free workplace where they can do homework. Create a predictable routine, and then experiment to see which specific background music works best with your child.

Chapter Six: Alternative or Supportive Treatments for ADHD

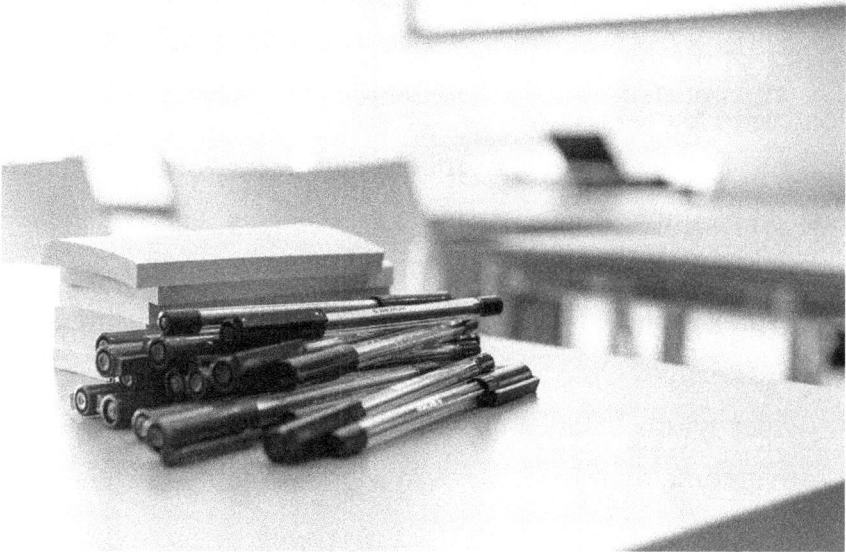

Many parents are understandably wary of medicating their children, and indeed many prefer behavioral therapies over medication. Or at the very least, behavioral therapy together with medication, rather than medication alone. Stimulants, for instance, may not be the best option for certain children - especially considering the possible side-effects and the long-term effects of drugs on a child's development. And because there is no such thing as a "cure" for ADHD - it is always a good idea to explore alternative therapies or treatments for ADHD, especially since it has been found that medication seems most effective when combined with other behavioral therapies rather than when medication alone is the preferred treatment.

There are a number of supportive treatments that can be implemented from home that can help the child manage their symptoms, without having to go to a professional. Helping the child through a nurturing and supportive home environment may actually provide the child with a balanced treatment plan that can help them overcome their difficulties in school or in their social lives.

In this chapter, we take a look at some of the simpler ways by which parents or families can help their children deal with and better manage the symptoms of ADHD. These must always be done in concert with professionally recommended treatments, however - whether therapy or medication. Always consult with your doctor before embarking on any alternative or home-based therapies.

Some Alternative Ways of Helping a Child Cope with ADHD

- Encouraging the child to exercise or to join a team sport

- Providing them with nutritious meals - learn how diet can affect the symptoms of ADHD

- Help the child de-stress by spending more time outdoors or in nature

- Establish predictable routines for meals, homework, play, and bed

- Help your child improve their social skills and social relationships

- Giving them rewards for small and big achievements

- Ensure that they get sufficient restful sleep

Exercise and spending time outdoors

Exercise is actually a natural way to achieve the same effects of stimulant medication - physical activity has been found to boost the brain's dopamine, norepinephrine, and serotonin levels - but without any of the side-effects.

Spending time in nature has also been found to reduce ADHD symptoms in children. Spending at least 30 minutes outdoors in nature daily can go a long way in helping your child manage the ADHD symptoms they are experiencing.

Joining or engaging in activities that involve physical exertion or movement, while at the same time also including a social component, can go a long way to helping your child manage their symptoms while at the same time improving their social skills. Encourage them to join extracurricular activities such as gymnastics, dance, martial arts, skateboarding, and team sports. Joining or engaging in practices such as yoga and tai-chi, which promote stillness and control, may also prove beneficial.

Regular quality sleep

One of the possible negative side-effects of stimulant medication is that it makes it difficult for the child to go to sleep at night. But a child needs regular quality sleep - in which case the dosage of the medication may be decreased or stopped altogether. Sleep is one of the best ways to ensure your child's continuing health, and regular quality sleep has been found to drastically improve ADHD symptoms.

If your child has difficulty going to sleep at night - with or without medication - you can help by ensuring an environment that promotes regular and restful sleep. Make sure that they go to bed at a regular time each night, eliminate all possible distractions from their bedroom such as TV's, games, phones at least an hour before bedtime. And finally, make sure that all physical activity during the evenings are limited so that your child is not too stimulated by the time they go to bed.

Good Nutrition

While food or food ingredients are not necessarily a cause of ADHD, feeding your child well and providing them with a nutritious and balanced diet can actually go a long way in helping your child manage some of the symptoms of ADHD. Some of the dietary changes you can implement from home include:

- Scheduling meals or snacks no more than three hours apart can help maintain their blood sugar level, while also minimizing irritability and supporting concentration and focus

- Omega-3 Fatty acids, which are found in salmon, tuna, sardines, and some fortified eggs and milk products, can help improve symptoms of hyperactivity and impulsivity in children. When approved by your doctor, you might also try giving them fish oil supplements to boost their supply of Omega-3 fatty acids.

- Boosting a child's zinc, iron and magnesium levels through dietary choices can go a long way in helping your child manage or improve their symptoms. For instance, iron supplements have been found to go a long way in improving the feelings restlessness among certain children.

- Protein and complex carbohydrates in your child's diet will help them feel more alert while also decreasing the levels of hyperactivity.

Techniques for Managing ADHD Symptoms for Adults

On the one hand, adults diagnosed with ADHD may have a more difficult time coping with the symptoms they are experiencing given the increased stresses and responsibilities of adult life. On the other hand, proper education and information regarding ADHD can go a long way in helping adults deal better with their condition - once they fully understand what they are going through, and why they need different ways of coping. Education, understanding, and acceptance, can be some of the first steps in helping adults with ADHD manage and improve their symptoms.

While medication is also an option for adults, this section focuses instead of some alternative techniques that any adult can implement to help them in better managing their symptoms.

- Find a supportive structure, whether among family, friends, or a support group. It makes a difference knowing that you are not alone in the struggles and difficulties that you face.

- Coaching can be extremely beneficial for some - by finding a coach who can encourage, remind you, and assist you as you try to implement various techniques in managing your symptoms. A level of trust, as well as a sense of humor, can prove quite beneficial from the right coach.

- Try to let go of negativity or guilt. It can be quite illuminating for some adults to learn that they have been suffering from undiagnosed ADHD all along. With this often comes a lifetime of guilt at not being able to meet social standards for relationships, work, or achievement, and even a sense that one was at fault or has done something wrong. Accepting the fact that your condition is a very real neuropsychiatric condition, and that it wasn't because you were lazy or less intelligent than others, can go a long way in helping you let go of a lifetime of baggage and negativity. Eventually, you must be able to let go of these past negative associations in order to successfully move forward in managing the symptoms you are experiencing.

- Find and experiment with various techniques that can help boost your performance at work - greater organizational skills and techniques, scheduling, color, coding, prioritizing, setting yourself goals and challenges, de-stressing and taking regular breaks, etc., will vary in their effects on people. Find the techniques that work for you, or adapt them to your own uses. You might be pleasantly surprised at how effectively doing these things can boost your work performance, and even improve your social relationships.

- Learn to deal with mood swings or bad moods, and how to navigate the ups and downs of daily emotional challenges. There will be feelings of joy and elation, just as there will also be feelings of loneliness and depression. The important thing is not to get too carried away by these mood changes. You might try giving yourself a time-out, spend time with friends, or even exercising regularly and vigorously may help. Exercise has been proven to be one of the most successful natural therapies for ADHD symptoms, and this is true for both children and adults.

- Try cultivating an interest in other people and in things outside of yourself. It is far too easy to look inward too much and berate oneself for our perceived flaws and weaknesses. Even when you already know that you have ADHD, the symptoms that you experience can often prove frustrating. By taking an interest in things outside of yourself, or by paying attention to the people around you, you may be able to find a better balance in your life. Sometimes, it isn't just about what's going on inside you, but also about what's going on with the world and with the people we care about.

Chapter Six: Alternative or Supportive Treatments for ADHD

Chapter Seven: The Future of ADHD

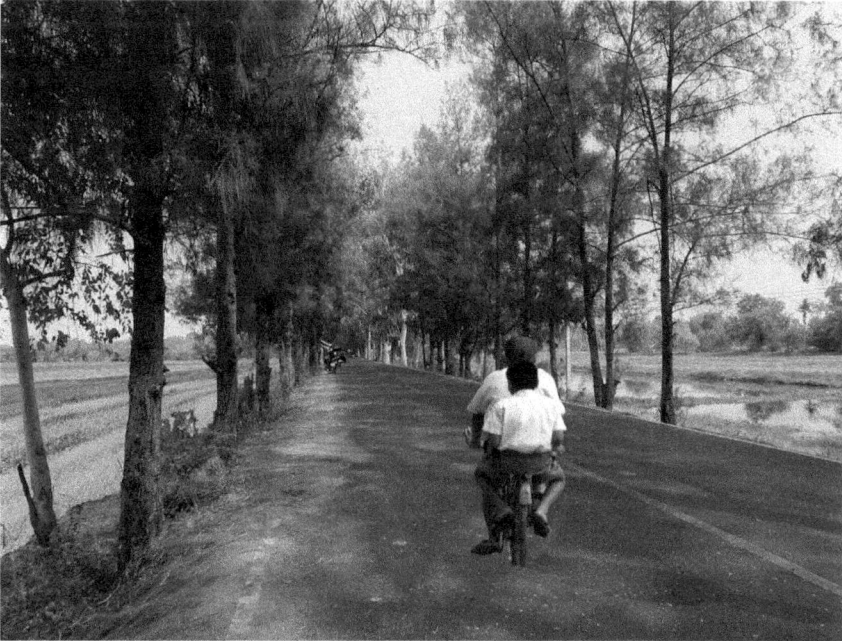

No, there is no "cure" for ADHD, and based on expert studies, ADHD symptoms are expected to last well into adulthood. Researchers, scientists are doctors are working hard not only to give us a better understanding of this condition, but also to provide us with advances and hopefully what will prove to be more successful treatments.

In this chapter, we take a look at some of the more recent developments in the field of ADHD studies and research.

A New Understanding of ADHD through Brain Imaging

Brain imaging is changing our way of understanding ADHD. These allow us to observe how the brain actually works, and what differences there may be with the brain functions of those without ADHD. This has already helped in bolstering the veracity of ADHD as "real mental condition" - in the face of very strong public sentiment that it isn't a real disease, but that it is all in one's head. Not only do brain imaging scans provide lend a verifiable veracity to all the ADHD studies and research, it also helps us to understand the condition a little bit better. Already, certain differences in brain functions, and even size have been noted between people with ADHD, and those without. What it all means has yet to be determined, however - at this point, the research is still too new. Hopefully, a better understanding of what ADHD is, what causes it, and how it works, will also enable us to produce more effective and lasting treatments.

Additional Research into ADHD

Certain moves are currently being undertaken to increase our research into ADHD. These include:

- Determining which combinations of ADHD treatment work best for different types of children. This is a 5-year study that is being cosponsored by NIMH and the U.S. Department of Education. It is hoped that the results of this research will help in more effective interventions and treatments.

- Research is also being conducted to determine whether or not there are different varieties of attention deficit. It is hoped that a number of different disorders may be covered by ADHD, each with its own symptoms and treatment requirements. These differences may also include slight physical differences that can help distinguish one type of ADHD from another.

- Further research is being conducted into the long-term effects or prognosis of ADHD, and what treatment methods undertaken during childhood can have the most impact during adulthood. It is hoped that this research can help in supporting the growth and development of children with ADHD into well-functioning adults.

It is also to be hoped that further research will also be conducted into adult ADHD. At this point, not much is still known about adult ADHD - and the lack of pertinent information can often be frustration. For instance:

- There is still a lack of consensus regarding the diagnostic tools to identify adult ADHD. Many feel that the symptoms in DSM-5 should also be adjusted to adults, and that an examination of past records - whether school or medical records - should also be included.

- It is also still not known to what extent the presence of comorbid disorders affects or influences the symptoms of ADHD. Having comorbid disorders may, in fact, cause greater confusion as to what precisely an adult is suffering from - whether it is simply depression, anxiety, bipolar disorder, or ADHD, or more than one at the same time. The difficulty is bolstered by the fact that many of the symptoms are similar between ADHD and other disorders. It is to be hoped that further research will throw some light on the effect of several disorders on each other, what differentiates them, what is the impact of their interaction on the individual, and which disorders and their respective symptoms should be targeted for treatment.

Prognosis for ADHD

The long-term prognosis for ADHD largely depends on our current efforts and understanding and treating this condition. Statistically, majority of children diagnosed with ADHD will continue having symptoms well into adulthood - but with proper treatment that should include behavioral therapy and coping and alternative strategies, the prognosis isn't too bad. In a way, with sufficient effort, the symptoms of ADHD can be manageable.

The important first step, of course, is awareness. There are many children with ADHD that have not yet been diagnosed, and around half of those who have been diagnosed do not have access to proper treatment methods. While there are many individuals and parents who claim that ADHD is not a real disorder, that it is overmedicated and over diagnosed, the truth is that better diagnostic tools that allow us to identify individuals suffering from ADHD can go a long way in giving them the help that they need. And given the long-term and serious effects of ADHD on a person's life, diagnosis and proper treatment is imperative if they are to be equipped with the tools to manage their condition.

With treatment, the prognosis can be good. Without treatment, however, we are looking at individuals going through life experiencing frustration and a higher risk of substance abuse, of getting into car accidents, and a potentially troubled life. The symptoms of ADHD can legitimately wreak havoc on an individual's familial and social relationships, not to mention their working and occupational lives.

No, there is still no cure for ADHD, but with proper knowledge, awareness, and sufficient support systems, its symptoms can be manageable.

Index

D

E

M

N

O

P

W

Photo References

Page 1 Photo by ProbenGammelmark via Pixabay. <https://pixabay.com/en/antique-classroom-desk-school-1854416/>

Page 5 Photo by isiddique via Pixabay. <https://pixabay.com/en/asia-classroom-nature-student-1675668/>

Page 21 Photo by U.S. Navy photo by Journalist 3rd Class Ryan C. McGinley via Wikimedia Commons. <https://commons.wikimedia.org/wiki/File:US_Navy_050222-N-3019M-001_Culinary_Specialist_1st_Class_Davidson_Cervantes,_assigned_to_the_guided_missile_frigate_USS_Crommelin_(FFG_37),_helps_a_child_read_a_book_at_Holomua_Elementary_School_in_Ewa_Beach,_Hawaii.jpg>

Page 31 Photo by markusspiske via Pixabay. <https://pixabay.com/en/board-child-school-children-learn-1666644/>

Page 39 Photo by The U.S Food and Drug Administration via Wikimedia Commons. <https://commons.wikimedia.org/wiki/File:How_Do_You

_Know_If_Your_Child_Has_ADHD%3F_(6348463190).jpg
>

Page 51 Photo by LaurMG. Via Wikimedia Commons.
<https://commons.wikimedia.org/wiki/File:Frustrated_ma
n_at_a_desk.jpg>

Page 61 Photo by Skitterphoto via Pixabay.
<https://pixabay.com/en/workshop-pens-post-it-note-
1746275/>

Page 71 Photo by likedok88 via Pixabay.
<https://pixabay.com/en/dear-students-the-group-people-
1593283/>

References

"9 Myths, Misconceptions and Stereotypes about ADHD." Margarita Tartakovsky, M.S. <http://psychcentral.com/blog/archives/2011/06/24/9-myths-misconceptions-and-stereotypes-about-adhd/>

"A Visual Guide to ADHD in Adults." WebMD. <http://www.webmd.com/add-adhd/ss/slideshow-adhd-in-adults>

"ADHD Across the Lifespan." myadhd. <http://www.myadhd.com/adhdacrosslifespan.html>

"ADHD Causes." Child Development Institute. <https://childdevelopmentinfo.com/add-adhd/adhd-causes/>

"ADHD: Inattentive Type." WebMD. <http://www.webmd.com/add-adhd/guide/adhd-inattentive-type#1>

"ADHD or ADD Treatment for Children." HelpGuide.org. <http://www.helpguide.org/articles/add-adhd/attention-deficit-disorder-adhd-treatment-in-children.htm>

"ADHD Treatment in Children." WebMD.
<http://www.webmd.com/add-adhd/adhd-treatment-overview>

"Adult ADHD: 50 Tips of Management." Dr. Hallowell.
<http://www.drhallowell.com/adult-adhd-50-tips-of-management/>

"Are There Really 7 Types of ADD?" ADDitude.
<http://www.additudemag.com/slideshow/61/slide-1.html>

"Attention-Deficit/Hyperactivity Disorder (ADHD)." CDC.
<http://www.cdc.gov/ncbddd/adhd/diagnosis.html>

"Attention Deficit Disorder ADD/ADHD." The Amen
Clinics. <http://danielamenmd.com/healthy-vs-unhealthy-2/attention-deficit-disorder-addadhd/>

"Attention Deficit Hyperactivity Disorder." National
Institute of Mental Health.
<https://www.nimh.nih.gov/health/topics/attention-deficit-hyperactivity-disorder-adhd/index.shtml>

"Attention deficit hyperactivity disorder." Wikipedia.
<https://en.wikipedia.org/wiki/Attention_deficit_hyperactivity_disorder>

"Attention Deficit Hyperactivity Disorder: Causes of ADHD." WebMD. <http://www.webmd.com/add-adhd/guide/adhd-causes>

"Attention Deficit Hyperactivity Disorder (ADHD) - Symptoms." NHS Choices. <http://www.nhs.uk/Conditions/Attention-deficit-hyperactivity-disorder/Pages/Symptoms.aspx>

"Attention-Deficit/Hyperactivity Disorder (ADHD) - Treatment." CDC. <http://www.cdc.gov/ncbddd/adhd/treatment.html>

"Attention deficit hyperactivty disorder (ADHD) - Treatment. NHS Choices. <http://www.nhs.uk/Conditions/Attention-deficit-hyperactivity-disorder/Pages/Treatment.aspx>

"Attention Deficit Hyperactivity Disorder (ADHD) Treatment & Management." Medscape. <http://emedicine.medscape.com/article/289350-treatment#d8>

"Causes of ADHD." myadhd. <http://www.myadhd.com/causesofadhd.html>

"Causes of ADHD: What We Know Today." healthychildren.org.

<https://www.healthychildren.org/English/health-issues/conditions/adhd/Pages/Causes-of-ADHD.aspx>

"Causes of Attention Deficit Disorder (ADHD)." Ben Martin, Psy. D. <http://psychcentral.com/lib/causes-of-attention-deficit-disorder-adhd/>

"Diagnostic Criteria for ADD/ADHD." David Rabiner, Ph.D. <http://www.helpforadd.com/criteria-for-add/>

"Dr. Amen's 7 Types of ADHD." Eve Kessler, Esq. <http://www.smartkidswithld.org/getting-help/adhd/7-types-adhd/>

"DSM-5TM." ADHD Institute. <http://www.adhd-institute.com/assessment-diagnosis/diagnosis/dsm-5tm/>

"Future Directions in ADHD." Everyday Health. <http://www.everydayhealth.com/adhd/adhd-research.aspx>

"Glossary of ADHD Terms." WebMD. <http://www.webmd.com/add-adhd/guide/adhd-glossary>

"Glossary of Terms Related to ADHD." National Resource Center on AD/HD. <http://209.126.179.230/en/about/Glossary>

"History of attention deficit hyperactivity disorder."
Wikipedia.
<https://en.wikipedia.org/wiki/History_of_attention_defi
cit_hyperactivity_disorder>

"Is it ADHD? Use our Checklist of Common Symptoms."
ADDitude.
<http://www.additudemag.com/adhd/article/621.html>

"Myths and Misunderstandings." National Resource Center
on AD/HD. <http://209.126.179.230/en/about/myths>

"New Diagnostic Criteria for ADHD: Subtle but Important
Changes." David Rabiner, Ph.D.
<http://www.helpforadd.com/2013/june.htm>

"Prognosis for ADHD in Children." Natasha Tracy.
<http://www.healthyplace.com/adhd/children-
behavioral-issues/prognosis-for-adhd-in-children/>

"Stimulant." Wikipedia.
<https://en.wikipedia.org/wiki/Stimulant>

"Symptoms and Diagnosis." ADHD Awareness Month.
<http://www.adhdawarenessmonth.org/symptoms-and-
diagnosis/>

"The 11 Biggest Myths and Misconceptions About Attention
Deficit Hyperactivity Disorder." Lecia Bushak.

<http://www.medicaldaily.com/11-biggest-myths-and-misconceptions-about-attention-deficit-hyperactivity-disorder-356008>

"The ADHD Prognosis is Promising." Diana Rodriquez. <http://www.everydayhealth.com/adhd/adhd-prognosis.aspx>

"The History of ADHD: A Timeline." HealthLine. <http://www.healthline.com/health/adhd/history#Overview1>

"The history of attention deficit hyperactivity disorder." Klaus W. Lange, Susanna Reichl, Katharina M. Lange, Lara Tucha, and Oliver Tucha. <https://www.ncbi.nlm.nih.gov/pmc/articles/PMC3000907/>

"Treatments for ADHD." myadhd. <http://www.myadhd.com/treatmentsforadhd.html>

"Types of ADHD." WebMD. <http://www.webmd.com/add-adhd/guide/types-of-adhd>

"Understanding ADHD - the Basics." WebMD. <http://www.webmd.com/add-adhd/childhood-adhd/understanding-adhd-basics>

"What Are the Possible Causes of ADHD?" ADHD & You. <http://www.adhdandyou.com/adhd-patient/what-is-adhd/causes-of-adhd.aspx>

"What Are the Three Types of ADHD?" Healthline. <http://www.healthline.com/health/adhd/three-types-adhd#Overview1>

"What Causes ADHD? 12 Myths and Facts." Kristin Koch. <http://www.health.com/health/gallery/0,,20441463,00.html>

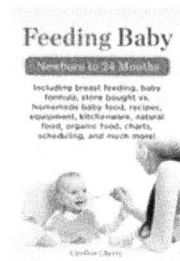

Feeding Baby
Cynthia Cherry
978-1941070000

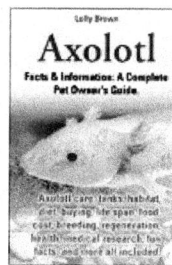

Axolotl
Lolly Brown
978-0989658430

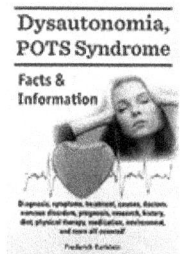

Dysautonomia, POTS
Syndrome
Frederick Earlstein
978-0989658485

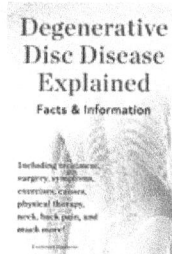

Degenerative Disc
Disease Explained
Frederick Earlstein
978-0989658485

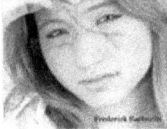

Sinusitis, Hay Fever,
Allergic Rhinitis Explained
Frederick Earlstein
978-1941070024

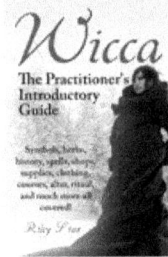

Wicca
Riley Star
978-1941070130

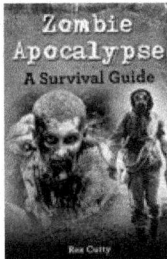

Zombie Apocalypse
Rex Cutty
978-1941070154

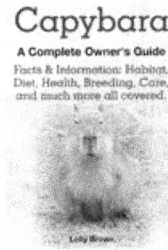

Capybara
Lolly Brown
978-1941070062

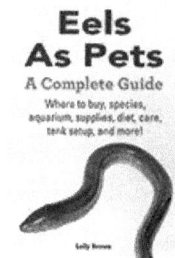

Eels As Pets
Lolly Brown
978-1941070167

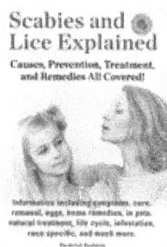

Scabies and Lice Explained
Frederick Earlstein
978-1941070017

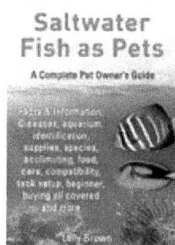

Saltwater Fish As Pets
Lolly Brown
978-0989658461

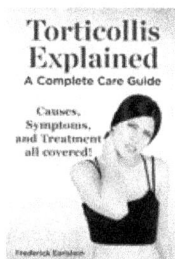

Torticollis Explained
Frederick Earlstein
978-1941070055

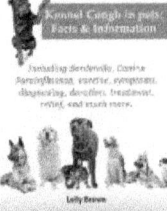

Kennel Cough
Lolly Brown
978-0989658409

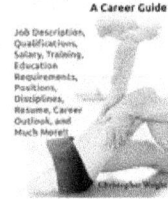

Physiotherapist, Physical
Therapist
Christopher Wright
978-0989658492

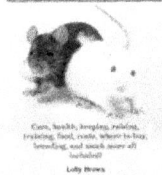

Rats, Mice, and Dormice
As Pets
Lolly Brown
978-1941070079

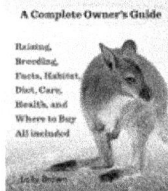

Wallaby and Wallaroo Care
Lolly Brown
978-1941070031

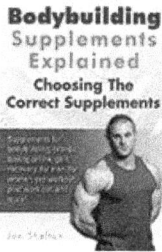

Bodybuilding Supplements
Explained
Jon Shelton
978-1941070239

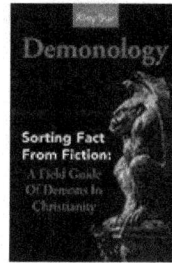

Demonology
Riley Star
978-19401070314

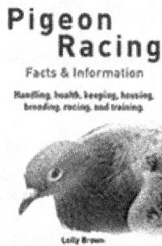

Pigeon Racing
Lolly Brown
978-1941070307

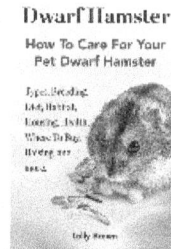

Dwarf Hamster
Lolly Brown
978-1941070390

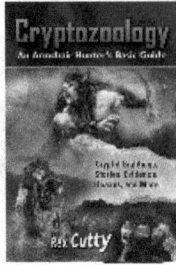

Cryptozoology
Rex Cutty
978-1941070406

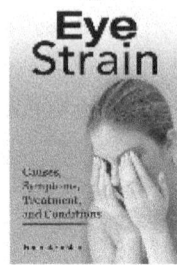

Eye Strain
Frederick Earlstein
978-1941070369

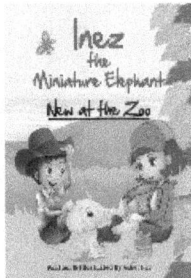

Inez The Miniature Elephant
Asher Ray
978-1941070353

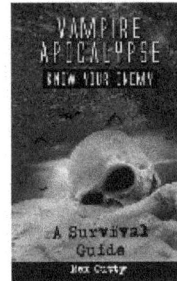

Vampire Apocalypse
Rex Cutty
978-1941070321

www.ingramcontent.com/pod-product-compliance
Lightning Source LLC
Chambersburg PA
CBHW060627210326
41520CB00010B/1500